Your Anti-Inflammatory Lifestyle Journal

six weeks of small changes to transform your body and mind

Julie Sochacki

"The best and most efficient pharmacy is within your own system." – Dr. Robert C. Peale

www.healedandthriving.com

ISBN: 978-0-9768599-1-8

Welcome!

Are you ready for 6 weeks of health coaching?

Whether your dream is to lose excess weight or just feel better in your body, complete a yoga class or a 5K, sit on the floor to play with children without pain or simply think more clearly, walk up a flight of stairs or crush it while playing tennis or golf: discover the power of mindful living with the *Your Anti-Inflammatory Lifestyle Journal*. This beautifully designed journal guides you to embrace habits that reduce inflammation and promote health, energy, and vitality. Inside, you'll find space to reflect on your daily choices, track anti-inflammatory foods, and celebrate your wins!

Learn to:

- Identify triggers that may contribute to inflammation.
- Embrace nourishing foods and lifestyle swaps.
- Enjoy improved sleep and stress-relief practices.
- Develop habits that support long-term well-being.

Whether you're beginning your health journey or deepening your practice, this journal is your companion for cultivating balance and reducing inflammation naturally.

Start today—your future self will thank you!

What is inflammation?

Inflammation is the body's natural response and a protective mechanism that helps the immune system heal and defend against damage. However, chronic inflammation is a prolonged, low-grade condition that can last for months or even years. It can be triggered by factors like stress, poor diet, or environmental factors. Over time, chronic inflammation will contribute to most health challenges. An anti-inflammatory lifestyle can reduce inflammation and support long-term vibrant health!

What are the benefits of an anti-inflammatory lifestyle?

Specifically, an anti-inflammatory lifestyle can reduce pain in the body, but it doesn't stop there. Significantly reducing inflammation can prevent and treat type two diabetes and keep blood sugar levels steady.

Research shows that an anti-inflammatory lifestyle also:

Reduces the risk of other chronic diseases like heart disease and cancer.

Improves joint health and reduces arthritis symptoms.

Enhances brain health and reduces cognitive decline.

Supports a healthy weight, reduces belly fat, and boosts metabolism.

Strengthens the immune system and reduces autoimmune flare-ups.

Improves digestive health and promotes a healthy gut microbiome.

Promotes skin health.

Improves longevity and quality of life.

Boosts energy levels.

Are you ready to feel better in your body?!

Let's simplify healthy eating.

Your food choices can either increase inflammation or decrease inflammation. In these transformative six weeks, you will have the opportunity to eliminate foods that are more likely to cause inflammation while adding foods that will begin to heal your body.

This journal empowers you to decide which foods to add each week based upon your preferences. **Choose whole foods and reduce and eliminate processed factory foods with simple food swaps.**

Choose organic whenever possible to reduce your exposure to glyphosate, an inflammatory chemical herbicide. Also, **choose foods with a lower glycemic index**, which support a slower rise in blood sugar levels.

Shortening your eating window supports an anti-inflammatory lifestyle. Notice how many hours you eat from start to finish each day. **Begin to move your eating into a 12 hour window.** Consider eating during daylight hours only. Feel free to enjoy water and black coffee and tea before your eating window begins.

Transform Your Plate: Anti-Inflammatory Food Swaps

Eat fresh real food and eliminate processed, factory foods.

Eat proteins like beans, lentils, fish, and lean meats. instead of processed meats like deli meats or sausage.

Eat fatty fish like wild-caught salmon, mackerel, cod, or sardines, which are high in omega-3 fatty acids.

Eat healthy fats like olive or avocado oil, rich in anti-inflammatory monounsaturated fats and antioxidants, instead of oils like soybean, corn, or canola oil. Choose olive oil over butter. When using butter choose grass-fed butter. Eat avocados, olives, nuts, and seeds.

Eat whole grains that regulate blood sugar like quinoa, rice and oats instead of grains that cause blood sugar to spike like white breads and wheat pasta. Try a lentil or bean pasta.

Eat fruits like berries, apples, and oranges, especially after meals, instead of sugary snacks.

Drink green tea or herbal teas instead of sugary beverages and alcohol.

Reduce or eliminate cheese, ice cream, and most dairy. Use unsweetened almond milk in moderation instead of dairy milk.

Transform Your Plate: Anti-Inflammatory Food Swaps

Eat roasted or steamed veggies instead of fried foods. Add mushrooms to your diet.

Eat fresh salads and increase veggies. Try fermented vegetables like sauerkraut and kimchi.

Eat Japanese sweet potatoes with white flesh, which can help regulate blood sugar, instead of white potatoes.

Eat natural sweeteners sparingly like honey or maple syrup, instead of white sugar. Enjoy dark chocolate, which is filled with polyphenols and have anti-inflammatory properties.

For an added benefit, add fresh and dried herbs and spices like turmeric (along with black pepper), cumin and curry powder (turmeric based), ginger, garlic, flat-leaf parsley, oregano, dill, chili peppers, basil, cinnamon, rosemary, thyme.

Note: Your body knows best. We are all different. These food swaps help most people to reduce inflammation. Sugar, dairy, and wheat could cause inflammation. If there is a swap that does not work for you, then concentrate on the ones that do.

Move your body!

Movement is a powerful tool in living an anti-inflammatory lifestyle—it reduces stress hormones, supports lymphatic flow, boosts circulation, and helps regulate immune function.

Movement plays a key role in reducing inflammation. Instead of committing to 30 minutes of exercise a day and being mostly sedentary for the other 23.5 hours of the day, move your body throughout the day.

Enjoy short bursts of movement like walk for 10 minutes, do chores around the house, cook a meal, wash the dog, meet a friend for a bike ride or for a game of tennis, roll out your Yoga mat and stretch your body.

Staying as active as you can throughout the day reduces inflammation. Add strength training for added benefits and ten minutes of movement after meals to regulate blood sugar.

Here's a go-to list of anti-inflammatory-friendly movements that are gentle on the joints, sustainable long-term, and super healing for the body and mind:

Walking (Especially in Nature)
Boosts circulation and lymph flow, and regulates cortisol (stress hormone)

Yoga (Gentle, Yin, or Restorative)
Reduces inflammation markers.

Stretching with Breath-Linked Movement (Pilates)
Focuses on breath and muscle activation

Strength Training (Bodyweight or Light Weights)
Helps reduce visceral fat (a major driver of inflammation)

Rebounding (Mini Trampoline)
Stimulates lymphatic drainage and helps move out toxins

Tai Chi or Qigong
Shown to lower inflammation and improve immune balance

Swimming or Aqua Aerobics
Gentle on joints, excellent for full-body movement

Dancing (Freeform or Structured)
Joyful movement lowers stress and inflammation

Improve Sleep!

When evaluating your sleep, it's important to focus on the quantity and quality of sleep. As far as the quantity of sleep, set yourself up for success by beginning a nighttime routine well before your 8 hours of sleep begins.

Leave electronic devices in the other room.

Keep your room dark and cool. Use black out curtains and sleep in the ideal temperature of 60–67°F (15–19°C).

Engage in a relaxing activity before bed like reading, meditating or drinking a cup of chamomile or lemon balm tea.

Evaluate your day, let go of all that you can, and then write down your best moment of the day. This simple practice will help you to quiet your mind once you close your eyes.

Get natural light early in the day to set your circadian rhythm.

Avoid late night eating and alcohol and caffeine intake.

Stick to a regular sleep schedule throughout the week.

Reduce stress!

We have a tendency to believe that we need to do more, not less. Instead of constantly doing, you have permission to just be. We are not human doings; we are human beings.

Consider meditating for 5 minutes a day or simply sit outside to get sun on your face.

Visit a beach, a park, or nature preserve to take a walk. Enjoy peaceful moments on your own or walk with a friend or pet to get the boosted benefits of connection.

Take a warm bath, listen to calm music, explore aromatherapy, read, or keep a gratitude journal.

Creating brings us joy--whether it's painting, singing, journaling or a DIY home project.

Taking digital detoxes with phone-free meals, unplugged Sundays, and screen-free evenings.

Forest bathing is the art of staying in the present moment to notice the beauty around you in nature. Also, "earthing" can be as simple as walking barefoot to connect with the Earth's natural electric charge. Finally, a practice of deep breathing can lower stress levels while oxygenating your blood.These practices decrease inflammation while increasing energy.

How to Use This Journal

Committing to a simple daily practice will help you to reduce inflammation.

1) Your job is to identify your lifestyle factors that cause inflammation and eliminate or at least reduce them.

2) You may also bring new practices into your life related to **nutrition, movement, sleep,** and **stress relief** that will further lower inflammation and improve all areas of your life!

There is one caveat: the key to transformation is having **self-compassion**. Like any new practice, some moments and decisions are better than others.

Consistency is more important than perfection. Think of this journal as your companion, as you embark on a new adventure towards improved health!

Use this QR Code (www.healedandthriving.com) to access a six week FREE course and become part of the Healed & Thriving Community!

Getting-Started Notes

Getting Started Survey

Date:__________

What are some possible foods that cause your inflammation now?

What movement do you get on a daily basis now?

Explain your quality and quantity of sleep now?

What do you do on a daily basis to reduce your stress level now?

Getting Started Survey

What are your symptoms of inflammation? (pain, fatigue, stomach issues, brain fog, headaches, mood changes, weight changes, etc.)

On a scale of 1-10 (1 being the lowest amount of pain or uncomfortableness and 10 being the most amount of pain or uncomfortableness), what is your pain level today?

____

Why do you want to make changes?

How motivated are you to take steps to improve your body and mind?

Daily Progress

Date:_________________

Anti-inflammatory foods you enjoyed today:

What was your eating window today?

__________ hours

(Calculate the hours from your first bite of food to your last. Water and black coffee and tea do not begin an eating window, because they likely don't spike blood sugar. Your target is a 12 hour eating window or less.)

Daily movement:

Today's sleep quantity:

_____ hours

Today's sleep quality:

_____ (ten (10) being the best night's sleep and one (1) being the worst)

Daily Progress

Today's stress-relief activities:

_____ total minutes

Best moment of the day:

On a scale of 1-10 (one (1) being the lowest amount of pain and ten (10) being the most amount of pain), what is your pain level today? ____________

What small steps can you take to decrease your inflammation tomorrow?

Daily Progress

Date:_______________

Anti-inflammatory foods you enjoyed today:

What was your eating window today?

__________ hours

(Calculate the hours from your first bite of food to your last. Water and black coffee and tea do not begin an eating window, because they likely don't spike blood sugar. Your target is a 12 hour eating window or less.)

Daily movement:

Today's sleep quantity:

_____ hours

Today's sleep quality:

_____ (ten (10) being the best night's sleep and one (1) being the worst)

Daily Progress

Today's stress-relief activities:

_____ total minutes

Best moment of the day:

On a scale of 1-10 (one (1) being the lowest amount of pain and ten (10) being the most amount of pain), what is your pain level today? ____________

What small steps can you take to decrease your inflammation tomorrow?

Daily Progress

Date:________________

Anti-inflammatory foods you enjoyed today:

What was your eating window today?

__________ hours

(Calculate the hours from your first bite of food to your last. Water and black coffee and tea do not begin an eating window, because they likely don't spike blood sugar. Your target is a 12 hour eating window or less.)

Daily movement:

Today's sleep quantity:

_____ hours

Today's sleep quality:

_____ (ten (10) being the best night's sleep and one (1) being the worst)

Daily Progress

Today's stress-relief activities:

_____ total minutes

Best moment of the day:

On a scale of 1-10 (one (1) being the lowest amount of pain and ten (10) being the most amount of pain), what is your pain level today? ____________

What small steps can you take to decrease your inflammation tomorrow?

Daily Progress

Date:__________________

Anti-inflammatory foods you enjoyed today:

What was your eating window today?

__________ hours

(Calculate the hours from your first bite of food to your last. Water and black coffee and tea do not begin an eating window, because they likely don't spike blood sugar. Your target is a 12 hour eating window or less.)

Daily movement:

Today's sleep quantity:

_____ hours

Today's sleep quality:

_____ (ten (10) being the best night's sleep and one (1) being the worst)

Daily Progress

Today's stress-relief activities:

_____ total minutes

Best moment of the day:

On a scale of 1-10 (one (1) being the lowest amount of pain and ten (10) being the most amount of pain), what is your pain level today? ____________

What small steps can you take to decrease your inflammation tomorrow?

Daily Progress

Date:__________________

Anti-inflammatory foods you enjoyed today:

What was your eating window today?

____________ hours

(Calculate the hours from your first bite of food to your last. Water and black coffee and tea do not begin an eating window, because they likely don't spike blood sugar. Your target is a 12 hour eating window or less.)

Daily movement:

Today's sleep quantity:

______ hours

Today's sleep quality:

______ (ten (10) being the best night's sleep and one (1) being the worst)

Daily Progress

Today's stress-relief activities:

_____ total minutes

Best moment of the day:

On a scale of 1-10 (one (1) being the lowest amount of pain and ten (10) being the most amount of pain), what is your pain level today? ______________

What small steps can you take to decrease your inflammation tomorrow?

Daily Progress

Date:________________

Anti-inflammatory foods you enjoyed today:

What was your eating window today?

__________ hours

(Calculate the hours from your first bite of food to your last. Water and black coffee and tea do not begin an eating window, because they likely don't spike blood sugar. Your target is a 12 hour eating window or less.)

Daily movement:

Today's sleep quantity:

_____ hours

Today's sleep quality:

_____ (ten (10) being the best night's sleep and one (1) being the worst)

Daily Progress

Today's stress-relief activities:

_____ total minutes

Best moment of the day:

On a scale of 1-10 (one (1) being the lowest amount of pain and ten (10) being the most amount of pain), what is your pain level today? _____________

What small steps can you take to decrease your inflammation tomorrow?

Daily Progress

Date:_________________

Anti-inflammatory foods you enjoyed today:

What was your eating window today?

___________ hours

(Calculate the hours from your first bite of food to your last. Water and black coffee and tea do not begin an eating window, because they likely don't spike blood sugar. Your target is a 12 hour eating window or less.)

Daily movement:

Today's sleep quantity:

_____ hours

Today's sleep quality:

_____ (ten (10) being the best night's sleep and one (1) being the worst)

Daily Progress

Today's stress-relief activities:

_____ total minutes

Best moment of the day:

On a scale of 1-10 (one (1) being the lowest amount of pain and ten (10) being the most amount of pain), what is your pain level today? ____________

What small steps can you take to decrease your inflammation tomorrow?

Weekly Progress

Date:

Share nutritional improvements from your week.

List two things related to nutrition and lifestyle (movement, sleep, and stress relief) that helped the most to decrease your inflammation and increase your wellness this week.

What small change can you celebrate this week? (increased movement, better sleep, less stress, feeling better overall)

Be specific!

How can you further reduce inflammation next week?

Prepare for Week 2

Daily Progress

Date:________________

Anti-inflammatory foods you enjoyed today:

What was your eating window today?

__________ hours

(Calculate the hours from your first bite of food to your last. Water and black coffee and tea do not begin an eating window, because they likely don't spike blood sugar. Your target is a 12 hour eating window or less.)

Daily movement:

Today's sleep quantity:

_____ hours

Today's sleep quality:

_____ (ten (10) being the best night's sleep and one (1) being the worst)

Daily Progress

Today's stress-relief activities:

_____ total minutes

Best moment of the day:

On a scale of 1-10 (one (1) being the lowest amount of pain and ten (10) being the most amount of pain), what is your pain level today? ______________

What small steps can you take to decrease your inflammation tomorrow?

Daily Progress

Date:_________________

Anti-inflammatory foods you enjoyed today:

What was your eating window today?

___________ hours

(Calculate the hours from your first bite of food to your last. Water and black coffee and tea do not begin an eating window, because they likely don't spike blood sugar. Your target is a 12 hour eating window or less.)

Daily movement:

Today's sleep quantity:

_____ hours

Today's sleep quality:

_____ (ten (10) being the best night's sleep and one (1) being the worst)

Daily Progress

Today’s stress-relief activities:

_____ total minutes

Best moment of the day:

On a scale of 1-10 (one (1) being the lowest amount of pain and ten (10) being the most amount of pain), what is your pain level today? _____________

What small steps can you take to decrease your inflammation tomorrow?

Daily Progress

Date:________________

Anti-inflammatory foods you enjoyed today:

What was your eating window today?

__________ hours

(Calculate the hours from your first bite of food to your last. Water and black coffee and tea do not begin an eating window, because they likely don't spike blood sugar. Your target is a 12 hour eating window or less.)

Daily movement:

Today's sleep quantity:

_____ hours

Today's sleep quality:

_____ (ten (10) being the best night's sleep and one (1) being the worst)

Daily Progress

Today's stress-relief activities:

_____ total minutes

Best moment of the day:

On a scale of 1-10 (one (1) being the lowest amount of pain and ten (10) being the most amount of pain), what is your pain level today? ____________

What small steps can you take to decrease your inflammation tomorrow?

Daily Progress

Date:________________

Anti-inflammatory foods you enjoyed today:

What was your eating window today?

__________ hours

(Calculate the hours from your first bite of food to your last. Water and black coffee and tea do not begin an eating window, because they likely don't spike blood sugar. Your target is a 12 hour eating window or less.)

Daily movement:

Today's sleep quantity:

_____ hours

Today's sleep quality:

_____ (ten (10) being the best night's sleep and one (1) being the worst)

Daily Progress

Today's stress-relief activities:

_____ total minutes

Best moment of the day:

On a scale of 1-10 (one (1) being the lowest amount of pain and ten (10) being the most amount of pain), what is your pain level today? ____________

What small steps can you take to decrease your inflammation tomorrow?

Daily Progress

Date:_________________

Anti-inflammatory foods you enjoyed today:

What was your eating window today?

__________ hours

(Calculate the hours from your first bite of food to your last. Water and black coffee and tea do not begin an eating window, because they likely don't spike blood sugar. Your target is a 12 hour eating window or less.)

Daily movement:

Today's sleep quantity:

_____ hours

Today's sleep quality:

_____ (ten (10) being the best night's sleep and one (1) being the worst)

Daily Progress

Today's stress-relief activities:

_____ total minutes

Best moment of the day:

On a scale of 1-10 (one (1) being the lowest amount of pain and ten (10) being the most amount of pain), what is your pain level today? ____________

What small steps can you take to decrease your inflammation tomorrow?

Daily Progress

Date:________________

Anti-inflammatory foods you enjoyed today:

What was your eating window today?

__________ hours

(Calculate the hours from your first bite of food to your last. Water and black coffee and tea do not begin an eating window, because they likely don't spike blood sugar. Your target is a 12 hour eating window or less.)

Daily movement:

Today's sleep quantity:

_____ hours

Today's sleep quality:

_____ (ten (10) being the best night's sleep and one (1) being the worst)

Daily Progress

Today’s stress-relief activities:

_____ total minutes

Best moment of the day:

On a scale of 1-10 (one (1) being the lowest amount of pain and ten (10) being the most amount of pain), what is your pain level today? ____________

What small steps can you take to decrease your inflammation tomorrow?

Daily Progress

Date:_______________

Anti-inflammatory foods you enjoyed today:

What was your eating window today?

__________ hours

(Calculate the hours from your first bite of food to your last. Water and black coffee and tea do not begin an eating window, because they likely don't spike blood sugar. Your target is a 12 hour eating window or less.)

Daily movement:

Today's sleep quantity:

_____ hours

Today's sleep quality:

_____ (ten (10) being the best night's sleep and one (1) being the worst)

Daily Progress

Today's stress-relief activities:

_____ total minutes

Best moment of the day:

On a scale of 1-10 (one (1) being the lowest amount of pain and ten (10) being the most amount of pain), what is your pain level today? _____________

What small steps can you take to decrease your inflammation tomorrow?

Weekly Progress

Date:

Share nutritional improvements from your week.

List two things related to nutrition and lifestyle (movement, sleep, and stress relief) that helped the most to decrease your inflammation and increase your wellness this week.

What small change can you celebrate this week? (increased movement, better sleep, less stress, feeling better overall)

Be specific!

How can you further reduce inflammation next week?

Prepare for Week 3

Daily Progress

Date:_______________

Anti-inflammatory foods you enjoyed today:

What was your eating window today?

__________ hours

(Calculate the hours from your first bite of food to your last. Water and black coffee and tea do not begin an eating window, because they likely don't spike blood sugar. Your target is a 12 hour eating window or less.)

Daily movement:

Today's sleep quantity:

_____ hours

Today's sleep quality:

_____ (ten (10) being the best night's sleep and one (1) being the worst)

Daily Progress

Today's stress-relief activities:

_____ total minutes

Best moment of the day:

On a scale of 1-10 (one (1) being the lowest amount of pain and ten (10) being the most amount of pain), what is your pain level today? ____________

What small steps can you take to decrease your inflammation tomorrow?

Daily Progress

Date:________________

Anti-inflammatory foods you enjoyed today:

What was your eating window today?

__________ hours

(Calculate the hours from your first bite of food to your last. Water and black coffee and tea do not begin an eating window, because they likely don't spike blood sugar. Your target is a 12 hour eating window or less.)

Daily movement:

Today's sleep quantity:

_____ hours

Today's sleep quality:

_____ (ten (10) being the best night's sleep and one (1) being the worst)

Daily Progress

Today's stress-relief activities:

_____ total minutes

Best moment of the day:

On a scale of 1-10 (one (1) being the lowest amount of pain and ten (10) being the most amount of pain), what is your pain level today? ____________

What small steps can you take to decrease your inflammation tomorrow?

Daily Progress

Date:________________

Anti-inflammatory foods you enjoyed today:

What was your eating window today?

__________ hours

(Calculate the hours from your first bite of food to your last. Water and black coffee and tea do not begin an eating window, because they likely don't spike blood sugar. Your target is a 12 hour eating window or less.)

Daily movement:

Today's sleep quantity:

_____ hours

Today's sleep quality:

_____ (ten (10) being the best night's sleep and one (1) being the worst)

Daily Progress

Today's stress-relief activities:

_____ total minutes

Best moment of the day:

On a scale of 1-10 (one (1) being the lowest amount of pain and ten (10) being the most amount of pain), what is your pain level today? ____________

What small steps can you take to decrease your inflammation tomorrow?

Daily Progress

Date:________________

Anti-inflammatory foods you enjoyed today:

What was your eating window today?

__________ hours

(Calculate the hours from your first bite of food to your last. Water and black coffee and tea do not begin an eating window, because they likely don't spike blood sugar. Your target is a 12 hour eating window or less.)

Daily movement:

Today's sleep quantity:

_____ hours

Today's sleep quality:

_____ (ten (10) being the best night's sleep and one (1) being the worst)

Daily Progress

Today's stress-relief activities:

_____ total minutes

Best moment of the day:

On a scale of 1-10 (one (1) being the lowest amount of pain and ten (10) being the most amount of pain), what is your pain level today? ____________

What small steps can you take to decrease your inflammation tomorrow?

Daily Progress

Date:________________

Anti-inflammatory foods you enjoyed today:

What was your eating window today?

__________ hours

(Calculate the hours from your first bite of food to your last. Water and black coffee and tea do not begin an eating window, because they likely don't spike blood sugar. Your target is a 12 hour eating window or less.)

Daily movement:

Today's sleep quantity:

_____ hours

Today's sleep quality:

_____ (ten (10) being the best night's sleep and one (1) being the worst)

Daily Progress

Today's stress-relief activities:

_____ total minutes

Best moment of the day:

On a scale of 1-10 (one (1) being the lowest amount of pain and ten (10) being the most amount of pain), what is your pain level today? ______________

What small steps can you take to decrease your inflammation tomorrow?

Daily Progress

Date:__________________

Anti-inflammatory foods you enjoyed today:

What was your eating window today?

___________ hours

(Calculate the hours from your first bite of food to your last. Water and black coffee and tea do not begin an eating window, because they likely don't spike blood sugar. Your target is a 12 hour eating window or less.)

Daily movement:

Today's sleep quantity:

_____ hours

Today's sleep quality:

_____ (ten (10) being the best night's sleep and one (1) being the worst)

Daily Progress

Today's stress-relief activities:

_____ total minutes

Best moment of the day:

On a scale of 1-10 (one (1) being the lowest amount of pain and ten (10) being the most amount of pain), what is your pain level today? ____________

What small steps can you take to decrease your inflammation tomorrow?

Daily Progress

Date:________________

Anti-inflammatory foods you enjoyed today:

What was your eating window today?

___________ hours

(Calculate the hours from your first bite of food to your last. Water and black coffee and tea do not begin an eating window, because they likely don't spike blood sugar. Your target is a 12 hour eating window or less.)

Daily movement:

Today's sleep quantity:

_____ hours

Today's sleep quality:

_____ (ten (10) being the best night's sleep and one (1) being the worst)

Daily Progress

Today's stress-relief activities:

_____ total minutes

Best moment of the day:

On a scale of 1-10 (one (1) being the lowest amount of pain and ten (10) being the most amount of pain), what is your pain level today? ____________

What small steps can you take to decrease your inflammation tomorrow?

Weekly Progress

Date:

Share nutritional improvements from your week.

List two things related to nutrition and lifestyle (movement, sleep, and stress relief) that helped the most to decrease your inflammation and increase your wellness this week.

What small change can you celebrate this week?
(increased movement, better sleep, less stress, feeling better overall)
Be specific!

How can you further reduce inflammation next week?

Prepare for Week 4

Daily Progress

Date:________________

Anti-inflammatory foods you enjoyed today:

What was your eating window today?

__________ hours

(Calculate the hours from your first bite of food to your last. Water and black coffee and tea do not begin an eating window, because they likely don't spike blood sugar. Your target is a 12 hour eating window or less.)

Daily movement:

Today's sleep quantity:

_____ hours

Today's sleep quality:

_____ (ten (10) being the best night's sleep and one (1) being the worst)

Daily Progress

Today's stress-relief activities:

_____ total minutes

Best moment of the day:

On a scale of 1-10 (one (1) being the lowest amount of pain and ten (10) being the most amount of pain), what is your pain level today? ____________

What small steps can you take to decrease your inflammation tomorrow?

Daily Progress

Date:_______________

Anti-inflammatory foods you enjoyed today:

What was your eating window today?

__________ hours

(Calculate the hours from your first bite of food to your last. Water and black coffee and tea do not begin an eating window, because they likely don't spike blood sugar. Your target is a 12 hour eating window or less.)

Daily movement:

Today's sleep quantity:

_____ hours

Today's sleep quality:

_____ (ten (10) being the best night's sleep and one (1) being the worst)

Daily Progress

Today's stress-relief activities:

_____ total minutes

Best moment of the day:

On a scale of 1-10 (one (1) being the lowest amount of pain and ten (10) being the most amount of pain), what is your pain level today? ____________

What small steps can you take to decrease your inflammation tomorrow?

Daily Progress

Date:________________

Anti-inflammatory foods you enjoyed today:

What was your eating window today?

__________ hours

(Calculate the hours from your first bite of food to your last. Water and black coffee and tea do not begin an eating window, because they likely don't spike blood sugar. Your target is a 12 hour eating window or less.)

Daily movement:

Today's sleep quantity:

_____ hours

Today's sleep quality:

_____ (ten (10) being the best night's sleep and one (1) being the worst)

Daily Progress

Today's stress-relief activities:

_____ total minutes

Best moment of the day:

On a scale of 1-10 (one (1) being the lowest amount of pain and ten (10) being the most amount of pain), what is your pain level today? ____________

What small steps can you take to decrease your inflammation tomorrow?

Daily Progress

Date:___________________

Anti-inflammatory foods you enjoyed today:

What was your eating window today?

___________ hours

(Calculate the hours from your first bite of food to your last. Water and black coffee and tea do not begin an eating window, because they likely don't spike blood sugar. Your target is a 12 hour eating window or less.)

Daily movement:

Today's sleep quantity:

_____ hours

Today's sleep quality:

_____ (ten (10) being the best night's sleep and one (1) being the worst)

Daily Progress

Today's stress-relief activities:

_____ total minutes

Best moment of the day:

On a scale of 1-10 (one (1) being the lowest amount of pain and ten (10) being the most amount of pain), what is your pain level today? ____________

What small steps can you take to decrease your inflammation tomorrow?

Daily Progress

Date:________________

Anti-inflammatory foods you enjoyed today:

What was your eating window today?

__________ hours

(Calculate the hours from your first bite of food to your last. Water and black coffee and tea do not begin an eating window, because they likely don't spike blood sugar. Your target is a 12 hour eating window or less.)

Daily movement:

Today's sleep quantity:

_____ hours

Today's sleep quality:

_____ (ten (10) being the best night's sleep and one (1) being the worst)

Daily Progress

Today's stress-relief activities:

_____ total minutes

Best moment of the day:

On a scale of 1-10 (one (1) being the lowest amount of pain and ten (10) being the most amount of pain), what is your pain level today? ____________

What small steps can you take to decrease your inflammation tomorrow?

Daily Progress

Date:________________

Anti-inflammatory foods you enjoyed today:

What was your eating window today?

__________ hours

(Calculate the hours from your first bite of food to your last. Water and black coffee and tea do not begin an eating window, because they likely don't spike blood sugar. Your target is a 12 hour eating window or less.)

Daily movement:

Today's sleep quantity:

_____ hours

Today's sleep quality:

_____ (ten (10) being the best night's sleep and one (1) being the worst)

Daily Progress

Today's stress-relief activities:

_____ total minutes

Best moment of the day:

On a scale of 1-10 (one (1) being the lowest amount of pain and ten (10) being the most amount of pain), what is your pain level today? ____________

What small steps can you take to decrease your inflammation tomorrow?

Daily Progress

Date:________________

Anti-inflammatory foods you enjoyed today:

What was your eating window today?

__________ hours

(Calculate the hours from your first bite of food to your last. Water and black coffee and tea do not begin an eating window, because they likely don't spike blood sugar. Your target is a 12 hour eating window or less.)

Daily movement:

Today's sleep quantity:

_____ hours

Today's sleep quality:

_____ (ten (10) being the best night's sleep and one (1) being the worst)

Daily Progress

Today's stress-relief activities:

_____ total minutes

Best moment of the day:

On a scale of 1-10 (one (1) being the lowest amount of pain and ten (10) being the most amount of pain), what is your pain level today? ____________

What small steps can you take to decrease your inflammation tomorrow?

Weekly Progress

Date:

Share nutritional improvements from your week.

List two things related to nutrition and lifestyle (movement, sleep, and stress relief) that helped the most to decrease your inflammation and increase your wellness this week.

What small change can you celebrate this week? (increased movement, better sleep, less stress, feeling better overall)

Be specific!

How can you further reduce inflammation next week?

Prepare for Week 5

Daily Progress

Date:__________________

Anti-inflammatory foods you enjoyed today:

What was your eating window today?

__________ hours

(Calculate the hours from your first bite of food to your last. Water and black coffee and tea do not begin an eating window, because they likely don't spike blood sugar. Your target is a 12 hour eating window or less.)

Daily movement:

Today's sleep quantity:

_____ hours

Today's sleep quality:

_____ (ten (10) being the best night's sleep and one (1) being the worst)

Daily Progress

Today's stress-relief activities:

_____ total minutes

Best moment of the day:

On a scale of 1-10 (one (1) being the lowest amount of pain and ten (10) being the most amount of pain), what is your pain level today? ____________

What small steps can you take to decrease your inflammation tomorrow?

Daily Progress

Date:________________

Anti-inflammatory foods you enjoyed today:

What was your eating window today?

__________ hours

(Calculate the hours from your first bite of food to your last. Water and black coffee and tea do not begin an eating window, because they likely don't spike blood sugar. Your target is a 12 hour eating window or less.)

Daily movement:

Today's sleep quantity:

_____ hours

Today's sleep quality:

_____ (ten (10) being the best night's sleep and one (1) being the worst)

Daily Progress

Today's stress-relief activities:

_____ total minutes

Best moment of the day:

On a scale of 1-10 (one (1) being the lowest amount of pain and ten (10) being the most amount of pain), what is your pain level today? ____________

What small steps can you take to decrease your inflammation tomorrow?

Daily Progress

Date:________________

Anti-inflammatory foods you enjoyed today:

What was your eating window today?

__________ hours

(Calculate the hours from your first bite of food to your last. Water and black coffee and tea do not begin an eating window, because they likely don't spike blood sugar. Your target is a 12 hour eating window or less.)

Daily movement:

Today's sleep quantity:

_____ hours

Today's sleep quality:

_____ (ten (10) being the best night's sleep and one (1) being the worst)

Daily Progress

Today's stress-relief activities:

_____ total minutes

Best moment of the day:

On a scale of 1-10 (one (1) being the lowest amount of pain and ten (10) being the most amount of pain), what is your pain level today? ____________

What small steps can you take to decrease your inflammation tomorrow?

Daily Progress

Date:________________

Anti-inflammatory foods you enjoyed today:

What was your eating window today?

__________ hours

(Calculate the hours from your first bite of food to your last. Water and black coffee and tea do not begin an eating window, because they likely don't spike blood sugar. Your target is a 12 hour eating window or less.)

Daily movement:

Today's sleep quantity:

_____ hours

Today's sleep quality:

_____ (ten (10) being the best night's sleep and one (1) being the worst)

Daily Progress

Today's stress-relief activities:

_____ total minutes

Best moment of the day:

On a scale of 1-10 (one (1) being the lowest amount of pain and ten (10) being the most amount of pain), what is your pain level today? ____________

What small steps can you take to decrease your inflammation tomorrow?

Daily Progress

Date:_________________

Anti-inflammatory foods you enjoyed today:

What was your eating window today?

___________ hours

(Calculate the hours from your first bite of food to your last. Water and black coffee and tea do not begin an eating window, because they likely don't spike blood sugar. Your target is a 12 hour eating window or less.)

Daily movement:

Today's sleep quantity:

_____ hours

Today's sleep quality:

_____ (ten (10) being the best night's sleep and one (1) being the worst)

Daily Progress

Today's stress-relief activities:

_____ total minutes

Best moment of the day:

On a scale of 1-10 (one (1) being the lowest amount of pain and ten (10) being the most amount of pain), what is your pain level today? ____________

What small steps can you take to decrease your inflammation tomorrow?

Daily Progress

Date:________________

Anti-inflammatory foods you enjoyed today:

What was your eating window today?

__________ hours

(Calculate the hours from your first bite of food to your last. Water and black coffee and tea do not begin an eating window, because they likely don't spike blood sugar. Your target is a 12 hour eating window or less.)

Daily movement:

Today's sleep quantity:

_____ hours

Today's sleep quality:

_____ (ten (10) being the best night's sleep and one (1) being the worst)

Daily Progress

Today's stress-relief activities:

_____ total minutes

Best moment of the day:

On a scale of 1-10 (one (1) being the lowest amount of pain and ten (10) being the most amount of pain), what is your pain level today? _____________

What small steps can you take to decrease your inflammation tomorrow?

Daily Progress

Date:____________________

Anti-inflammatory foods you enjoyed today:

What was your eating window today?

__________ hours

(Calculate the hours from your first bite of food to your last. Water and black coffee and tea do not begin an eating window, because they likely don't spike blood sugar. Your target is a 12 hour eating window or less.)

Daily movement:

Today's sleep quantity:

_____ hours

Today's sleep quality:

_____ (ten (10) being the best night's sleep and one (1) being the worst)

Daily Progress

Today's stress-relief activities:

_____ total minutes

Best moment of the day:

On a scale of 1-10 (one (1) being the lowest amount of pain and ten (10) being the most amount of pain), what is your pain level today? ____________

What small steps can you take to decrease your inflammation tomorrow?

Weekly Progress

Date:

Share nutritional improvements from your week.

List two things related to nutrition and lifestyle (movement, sleep, and stress relief) that helped the most to decrease your inflammation and increase your wellness this week.

What small change can you celebrate this week? (increased movement, better sleep, less stress, feeling better overall)

Be specific!

How can you further reduce inflammation next week?

Prepare for Week 6

Daily Progress

Date:________________

Anti-inflammatory foods you enjoyed today:

What was your eating window today?

__________ hours

(Calculate the hours from your first bite of food to your last. Water and black coffee and tea do not begin an eating window, because they likely don't spike blood sugar. Your target is a 12 hour eating window or less.)

Daily movement:

Today's sleep quantity:

_____ hours

Today's sleep quality:

_____ (ten (10) being the best night's sleep and one (1) being the worst)

Daily Progress

Today's stress-relief activities:

_____ total minutes

Best moment of the day:

On a scale of 1-10 (one (1) being the lowest amount of pain and ten (10) being the most amount of pain), what is your pain level today? _____________

What small steps can you take to decrease your inflammation tomorrow?

Daily Progress

Date:_______________

Anti-inflammatory foods you enjoyed today:

What was your eating window today?

__________ hours

(Calculate the hours from your first bite of food to your last. Water and black coffee and tea do not begin an eating window, because they likely don't spike blood sugar. Your target is a 12 hour eating window or less.)

Daily movement:

Today's sleep quantity:

_____ hours

Today's sleep quality:

_____ (ten (10) being the best night's sleep and one (1) being the worst)

Daily Progress

Today’s stress-relief activities:

_____ total minutes

Best moment of the day:

On a scale of 1-10 (one (1) being the lowest amount of pain and ten (10) being the most amount of pain), what is your pain level today? ____________

What small steps can you take to decrease your inflammation tomorrow?

Daily Progress

Date:_______________

Anti-inflammatory foods you enjoyed today:

What was your eating window today?

__________ hours

(Calculate the hours from your first bite of food to your last. Water and black coffee and tea do not begin an eating window, because they likely don't spike blood sugar. Your target is a 12 hour eating window or less.)

Daily movement:

Today's sleep quantity:

_____ hours

Today's sleep quality:

_____ (ten (10) being the best night's sleep and one (1) being the worst)

Daily Progress

Today's stress-relief activities:

_____ total minutes

Best moment of the day:

On a scale of 1-10 (one (1) being the lowest amount of pain and ten (10) being the most amount of pain), what is your pain level today? ____________

What small steps can you take to decrease your inflammation tomorrow?

Daily Progress

Date:__________________

Anti-inflammatory foods you enjoyed today:

What was your eating window today?

__________ hours

(Calculate the hours from your first bite of food to your last. Water and black coffee and tea do not begin an eating window, because they likely don't spike blood sugar. Your target is a 12 hour eating window or less.)

Daily movement:

Today's sleep quantity:

_____ hours

Today's sleep quality:

_____ (ten (10) being the best night's sleep and one (1) being the worst)

Daily Progress

Today's stress-relief activities:

_____ total minutes

Best moment of the day:

On a scale of 1-10 (one (1) being the lowest amount of pain and ten (10) being the most amount of pain), what is your pain level today? ____________

What small steps can you take to decrease your inflammation tomorrow?

Daily Progress

Date:________________

Anti-inflammatory foods you enjoyed today:

What was your eating window today?

__________ hours

(Calculate the hours from your first bite of food to your last. Water and black coffee and tea do not begin an eating window, because they likely don't spike blood sugar. Your target is a 12 hour eating window or less.)

Daily movement:

Today's sleep quantity:

_____ hours

Today's sleep quality:

_____ (ten (10) being the best night's sleep and one (1) being the worst)

Daily Progress

Today’s stress-relief activities:

_____ total minutes

Best moment of the day:

On a scale of 1-10 (one (1) being the lowest amount of pain and ten (10) being the most amount of pain), what is your pain level today? _____________

What small steps can you take to decrease your inflammation tomorrow?

Daily Progress

Date:__________________

Anti-inflammatory foods you enjoyed today:

What was your eating window today?

__________ hours

(Calculate the hours from your first bite of food to your last. Water and black coffee and tea do not begin an eating window, because they likely don't spike blood sugar. Your target is a 12 hour eating window or less.)

Daily movement:

Today's sleep quantity:

_____ hours

Today's sleep quality:

_____ (ten (10) being the best night's sleep and one (1) being the worst)

Daily Progress

Today's stress-relief activities:

_____ total minutes

Best moment of the day:

On a scale of 1-10 (one (1) being the lowest amount of pain and ten (10) being the most amount of pain), what is your pain level today? _____________

What small steps can you take to decrease your inflammation tomorrow?

Daily Progress

Date:________________

Anti-inflammatory foods you enjoyed today:

What was your eating window today?

__________ hours

(Calculate the hours from your first bite of food to your last. Water and black coffee and tea do not begin an eating window, because they likely don't spike blood sugar. Your target is a 12 hour eating window or less.)

Daily movement:

Today's sleep quantity:

_____ hours

Today's sleep quality:

_____ (ten (10) being the best night's sleep and one (1) being the worst)

Daily Progress

Today's stress-relief activities:

_____ total minutes

Best moment of the day:

On a scale of 1-10 (one (1) being the lowest amount of pain and ten (10) being the most amount of pain), what is your pain level today? ____________

What small steps can you take to decrease your inflammation tomorrow?

Weekly Progress

Date:

Share nutritional improvements from your week.

List two things related to nutrition and lifestyle (movement, sleep, and stress relief) that helped the most to decrease your inflammation and increase your wellness this week.

What small change can you celebrate this week? (increased movement, better sleep, less stress, feeling better overall)

Be specific!

How can you further reduce inflammation next week?

Big Takeaways

Final Survey

Date:______________

What are your favorite foods that improved your overall health over the past six weeks?

What movement do you enjoy on a daily basis now?

Explain your quality and quantity of sleep now?

What do you do on a daily basis to reduce your stress level now?

Final Survey

What are your current symptoms of inflammation?

On a scale of 1-10 (one (1) being the lowest amount of pain and ten (10) being the most amount of pain), what is your pain level today? _______

What motivates you to keep going?

List some next steps to continue to see results.

How will you celebrate your positive changes?

References

Aly S. M. (2014). Role of intermittent fasting on improving health and reducing diseases. *International journal of health sciences, 8*(3), V–VI.

Fiuza-Luces, C., Santos-Lozano, A., Joyner, M., Carrera-Bastos, P., Picazo, O., Zugaza, J. L., Izquierdo, M., Ruilope, L. M., & Lucia, A. (2018). Exercise benefits in cardiovascular disease: beyond attenuation of traditional risk factors. *Nature reviews. Cardiology, 15*(12), 731–743.

Itsiopoulos, C., Mayr, H. L., & Thomas, C. J. (2022). The anti-inflammatory effects of a Mediterranean diet: a review. *Current opinion in clinical nutrition and metabolic care, 25*(6), 415–422.

Luo, B., Xiang, D., Ji, X., Chen, X., Li, R., Zhang, S., Meng, Y., Nieman, D. C., & Chen, P. (2024). The anti-inflammatory effects of exercise on autoimmune diseases: A 20-year systematic review. *Journal of sport and health science, 13*(3), 353–367.

Pascoe, M. C., Thompson, D. R., Jenkins, Z. M., & Ski, C. F. (2017). Mindfulness mediates the physiological markers of stress: Systematic review and meta-analysis. *Journal of psychiatric research, 95*, 156–178.

Stromsnes, K., Correas, A. G., Lehmann, J., Gambini, J., & Olaso-Gonzalez, G. (2021). Anti-Inflammatory Properties of Diet: Role in Healthy Aging. *Biomedicines, 9*(8), 922.

van Zonneveld, S. M., van den Oever, E. J., Haarman, B. C. M., Grandjean, E. L., Nuninga, J. O., van de Rest, O., & Sommer, I. E. C. (2024). An Anti-Inflammatory Diet and Its Potential Benefit for Individuals with Mental Disorders and Neurodegenerative Diseases-A Narrative Review. *Nutrients, 16*(16), 2646.

Zhao, M., Tuo, H., Wang, S., & Zhao, L. (2020). The Effects of Dietary Nutrition on Sleep and Sleep Disorders. *Mediators of inflammation, 2020*, 3142874.

Julie Sochacki is the heart and soul behind the research-based Healed and Thriving Journals. As a functional medicine certified health coach; a life-long learner, an educator and college professor; a whole-foods plant-based home cook; and a 200-hour Kripalu certified yoga teacher, Julie's mission is to empower and inspire everyone to prioritize small actionable steps that lead to wellness, healing, and thriving.

Go to **www.healedandthriving.com** to access the FREE six-week course!

Let Julie continue to inspire, motivate and empower you on your journey!

Made in United States
Orlando, FL
11 November 2026

90609394R00066